What Is Depression?

Major depressive disorder, also referred to here as *depression,* is a serious medical illness that disrupts a person's mood, behavior, thought processes, and physical health. Major depressive disorder should not be mistaken for the passing feelings of unhappiness that everyone experiences, nor should it be confused with the intense grief brought about by the death of a loved one. Sadness and grief are normal reactions to life stresses. With time, and usually without medical treatment, sadness and grief lift, and people go on with their lives. By contrast, without specialized medical treatment, depression often persists. But with effective treatment, a large majority of people improve significantly.

In most instances, major depressive disorder is a recurrent, episodic illness. This means that a person who has been depressed once and has recovered is likely to have one or more episodes of depression in the future, often within 2 to 3 years.

When depression is not treated, or is treated inappropriately, it is potentially fatal: nearly one in six people with severe, untreated depression commits suicide. However, seeking help and receiving an accurate diagnosis from a psychiatrist or other health care professional is a crucial and often decisive step toward recovery.

Many people with major depressive disorder do not recognize that they are ill. They, and others around them, may consider depression a sign of personal weakness. Some depressed people, faulting themselves for having the moods and feelings associated with their illness, purposely do not seek medical help. The symptoms experienced in depression are not a cause for shame, but a signal that medical help is needed. Doctors in all medical specialties are becoming more and more aware that depression is a commonplace, serious, and real illness. The course of an episode of major depressive disorder is predictable, and there are many treatments that address different aspects of the illness and, in the vast majority of cases, produce a positive effect.

Major depressive disorder is one form of depressive illness, or mood disorder. Other forms include bipolar disorder (manic-depressive illness) and dysthymia. In *bipolar disorder,* episodes of depression alternate with episodes of *mania,* a condition in which inappropriate or extreme "high" feelings may lead to dangerous, destructive behavior. *Dysthymia* involves symptoms similar to those of major depressive disorder. The symptoms are milder but longer lasting, and although they might not be disabling, they prevent a person from feeling good or operating at "full steam." Occasionally, a person with dysthymia may also have major depressive disorder, a condition referred to as *double depression*. This guide focuses on major depressive disorder.

What Are the Signs and Symptoms of Depression?

Depression is sometimes difficult to recognize because many of the *signs* that are noticeable by other people and the *symptoms* that a patient experiences differ only subtly from people's normal sensations and reactions. But many years of research, and also of observation by psychiatrists who work directly with patients, suggest that there is a specific set of signs and symptoms that indicate major depressive disorder. These include the following:

▶ A loss of interest in activities that normally are pleasurable, including sex

▶ Appetite and weight changes (either loss or gain)

▶ Sleep disturbances (insomnia, early morning wakening, or oversleeping)

▶ Feelings of guilt, worthlessness, or helplessness

▶ Feelings of hopelessness or pessimism

▶ Difficulty in concentrating, remembering, or making decisions

▶ Thoughts of death or suicide; suicide attempts

▶ Persistent body aches and pains or digestive disorders not caused by physical disease

Anyone who experiences five or more of these symptoms for at least 2 weeks may have a depressive illness and should seek the advice and assistance of a psychiatrist or other doctor.

Who Gets Depression?

Depression is one of the most frequently occurring mental illnesses. In any 6-month period, nearly 6% of adults in the United States have depression. Unlike other depressive illnesses (such as bipolar disorder) that affect men and women equally, major depressive disorder occurs about twice as often in women as in men. Depression affects people of all ages, but the illness most commonly first appears during a person's late twenties. High rates of depression are seen in very elderly people.

The risk of depression varies among certain individuals and groups. The children, brothers and sisters, and parents of a person with major depressive disorder are up to three times more likely to have the illness than are people with no history of depression in their families. People with chronic general medical illnesses (that is, physical illnesses) and those with drug and alcohol abuse disorders are also at higher than average risk.

What Causes Depression?

Major depressive disorder is not caused by any single factor. Researchers now believe that it is a result of genetic, biological, and psychological influences combined with life stresses. Disturbances in brain biochemistry (the chemicals in the brain and how they work) are an important factor in depression. Irregularities in specific brain chemicals, called *neurotransmitters,* occur in depression as well as in other mental illnesses. Scientists are now examining which of these irregularities may *cause* depression and which are a *result* of the illness.

Difficult life events, such as problem relationships, money difficulties, or the loss of a loved one, appear to contribute to depression. Sometimes depression is associated with a general medical illness. Drinking too much alcohol or using drugs can also lead to depression. Certain personality characteristics—such as pessimistic thinking, low self-esteem, and a sense of having little control over life events—have been linked to a vulnerability to depression. However, major depressive disorder is not caused by personal weakness or a lack of willpower.

How Is Depression Treated?

Diagnosis

The first step in treating depression is a thorough diagnostic evaluation. Mild to moderate depression can be diagnosed and treated by a general medical doctor, but patients who have severe depression—with or without other psychiatric disorders—and those who do not respond adequately to treatment should be evaluated and treated by a psychiatrist. The diagnostic evaluation includes

▶ A review of the signs and symptoms listed on page 2

▶ A physical examination, which includes a neurological examination (checking a patient's coordination, reflexes, balance, and other neurological functions to make sure that there are no other brain disorders), and laboratory tests

▶ A thorough medical and psychiatric history, including all current treatments and responses to previous treatments

The physical examination and laboratory tests can rule out disorders that produce symptoms similar to those found in a depressive illness—disorders such as thyroid disease, anemia, or a recent viral infection. On occasion, an electroencephalogram (EEG) or a brain scan will be done to get information about the structure of the brain and how it is functioning.

Knowledge about the occurrence of psychiatric disorders, especially depressive illnesses, among other family members aids in the choice of treatment approaches. This information may also suggest the future course of the patient's immediate illness. If there is a family history of recurrent depression, for example, it is more likely that a patient's depression will recur. Another example: a family history of bipolar disorder suggests the need for caution in the use of antidepressant medications. Some patients with major depressive disorder may have hidden bipolar disorder that can be triggered by antidepressant medications.

Treatment Setting

Most depressed patients can be treated as outpatients, either in a doctor's office or in an outpatient clinic. In some instances, however, a patient may require a brief period of hospitalization. Inpatient care and careful medical monitoring may be necessary when an episode of depression is

▶ Particularly severe and accompanied by serious weight loss or marked agitation

▶ Accompanied by intent to harm self or others

or

▶ So incapacitating that a patient cannot perform self-care, follow the doctor's instructions, or describe feelings to the doctor

It also may be best to hospitalize

▶ A patient who lacks supportive relationships or access to constructive activities

or

▶ A patient who may engage in dangerous activities, such as alcohol or illicit drug use

During hospitalizations, careful evaluations can be done, the patient can be detoxified from illicit drugs or alcohol, the patient can be protected, and intensive treatments can begin.

Treatment Plan

A treatment plan for depression consists of three distinct phases (also see the table "Treatment Phases and Goals" on the next page):

▶ Phase 1, *acute treatment,* relieves the immediate symptoms of depression.

▶ Phase 2, *continuation treatment,* preserves the gains achieved initially and protects the patient from sliding back into depression.

▶ Phase 3, *maintenance treatment,* guards against future episodes.

The following sections explain each phase and treatment during that phase.

Acute Phase

Several different approaches are highly effective in treating depression. These approaches fall into two general categories:

Treatment Phases and Goals		
Phase	**Length**	**Treatment goal**
Acute	6–8 weeks	Achieve remission
Continuation	16–20 weeks	Prevent relapse
Maintenance	Varies	Protect against recurrence

Remission = return to level of symptoms and functioning that existed before illness.
Relapse = re-emergence of significant depressive symptoms.
Recurrence = another major depressive episode.

▶ Somatic, or physical, treatments (including antidepressant medications, electroconvulsive therapy [ECT], and light therapy)

▶ Various types of psychotherapy

In choosing among the various approaches, the treating clinician considers

▶ The severity and stage of the illness

▶ The pattern of symptoms

▶ How well the patient is able to cope with the challenge of illness, especially whether the patient shows any signs of vulnerability to suicide

▶ A patient's preferences about treatment

▶ The cost of different approaches

▶ The availability of clinicians with appropriate training and expertise in specific types of psychotherapy

Antidepressant Medications

Antidepressant medications remedy chemical imbalances in the brain that are associated with major depressive disorder. Three classes of antidepressant medication currently available are

▶ Cyclic antidepressants

▶ Monoamine oxidase inhibitors (MAOIs)

▶ Selective serotonin reuptake inhibitors (SSRIs)

(See the "Antidepressant Medications" table on the next page for a list of drug names.) All antidepressants can take away or reduce the symptoms of depression and help a person return to feeling as he or she did before becoming depressed.

Each medication acts differently and has different side effects. Moreover, different individuals may respond differently to the same medication. Overall, however, more than two out of three patients benefit from antidepressant medication.

Although a patient will usually feel better within a week or two—experiencing, for example, improved sleep patterns or fewer physical complaints—a full appraisal of how well a medication is working requires 6 to 8 weeks. Weekly doctor visits are enough in most cases for monitoring the patient's response to treatment, the development of side effects, and the safety of the medication for the patient. In complex cases, the patient may need to meet with the doctor several times a week.

All antidepressant medications currently available are similar in their effectiveness. Therefore, choosing which medication to start with is usually based on the following:

▶ Anticipated side effects

▶ Safety or tolerability of these side effects for a particular patient

▶ Patient preference

▶ History of prior response to a medication

▶ Potential interactions with other medications a patient is taking

▶ Cost

▶ Presence of other psychiatric or general medical conditions

Side effects. Generally, the side effects of the newer antidepressants are fewer and less difficult to tolerate than the side effects of the older (cyclic) antidepressants. (Newer antidepressants include the SSRIs and some others such as *bupropion* and *trazodone*.)

Antidepressant Medications

Class	Generic name	Selected trade names
Cyclic antidepressants	Amitriptyline	Elavil, Endep
	Amoxapine	Asendin
	Clomipramine	Anafranil
	Desipramine	Norpramin, Pertofrane
	Doxepin	Adapin, Sinequan
	Imipramine	Tofranil, SK-Pramine
	Maprotiline	Ludiomil
	Nortriptyline	Pamelor
	Protriptyline	Vivactil
	Trimipramine	Surmontil
Monoamine oxidase inhibitors (MAOIs)	Isocarboxazid	Marplan
	Phenelzine	Nardil
	Tranylcypromine	Parnate
Selective serotonin reuptake inhibitors (SSRIs)	Citalopram	Celexa
	Fluoxetine	Prozac
	Fluvoxamine	Luvox
	Paroxetine	Paxil
	Sertraline	Zoloft
Other antidepressants	Bupropion	Wellbutrin
	Mirtazapine	Remeron
	Nefazodone	Serzone
	Reboxetine	Vestra
	Trazodone	Desyrel
	Venlafaxine	Effexor

Possible side effects of cyclic antidepressants include blurred vision, dry mouth, constipation, difficulty urinating, changes in sexual desire or ability, weight gain, muscle twitches, increased heart rate, low blood pressure and dizziness, and sedation.

Possible side effects of SSRIs include nausea, vomiting, diarrhea, restlessness, agitation, sleep disturbances, problems with sexual functioning, headaches, and temporary weight loss.

Possible side effects of MAOIs include low blood pressure, weight gain, problems with sexual functioning, headaches, and insomnia.

In addition, MAOIs can be associated with a severe reaction called a *hypertensive crisis*. It may occur if a patient taking an MAOI consumes food or medicine containing tyramine (see below). The hypertensive crisis is characterized by sudden onset of severe headache, nausea, neck stiffness, rapid heartbeat, increased sweating, and confusion. A hypertensive crisis may lead to a stroke or death. Because of this possible reaction, MAOIs are generally used only for patients who do not respond to or who cannot tolerate other antidepressant medications. Patients who take MAOIs need to follow strict dietary restrictions. These include avoiding tyramine-containing foods such as aged cheeses or meats, fermented products, yeast extracts, fava or broad beans, and overripe or spoiled foods. Medicines to be avoided include over-the-counter decongestants and cold remedies.

Not all the medications in these classes produce all these effects, and not all people experience them. Some side effects, such as the sedation associated with cyclic antidepressants and the nausea and vomiting that may occur with the SSRIs, disappear soon after a patient begins taking a medication. Others may remain throughout treatment. Patients should discuss all side effects with their doctors.

Sometimes the solution to a side effect may be simple—for example, taking a medication at bedtime to lessen problems caused by sedation, using sugarless gum or candy to relieve dry mouth, or drinking more water and eating more fiber to relieve constipation. Sometimes, however, it may be necessary to change the dose or, if problems are intolerable, to switch to a different medication.

Dosing. In selecting and adjusting the dose of a medication, the doctor takes into consideration the full range of side effects associated with a medication, the typically effective dose range, and the patient's age and health status. Usually, the patient will begin taking a medication at lower than the standard dose. The doctor will then gradually increase the dose until it reaches an effective level.

An overdose of antidepressant medications—especially the older cyclics—is serious and potentially lethal. Although antidepressants should decrease, rather than increase, the risk of suicidal thoughts and behaviors, some patients may become suicidal after treatment begins. Patients who find themselves dwelling on suicide or experiencing impulses to harm themselves should talk about it with their doctor.

Psychotherapy

Psychotherapy comes in many variations and is offered for groups, families, couples, and individuals. Common to all forms of psychotherapy is a patient's talking with a therapist. A variety of therapies are designed specifically to help a person gain insight into factors that may have contributed to depression or may be maintaining it. Problems are discussed and resolved through the insights, understanding, and emotional support gained from verbal give-and-take. A therapist is likely to draw elements from several psychotherapeutic approaches, depending on the individual's needs and interests. As in treatment with medications, the frequency of visits during psychotherapy varies, depending on the complexity of the depression, from once a week to several times a week.

Psychodynamic approaches are based on the assumption that internal psychological conflicts are major factors in an individual's depression. (For example, a person may want to be both independent and cared for; another person may feel angry while believing that one should always be kind and loving.) Successful treatment depends on being able to resolve these conflicts, which often are rooted in early childhood. The aim of treatment is to bring the conflict into the open, where it can be resolved by the patient with the insights of the therapist.

Interpersonal therapy focuses on current conflicts and interpersonal problems. This therapy alone may be effective in treating mild forms of depression that do not have substantial physical symptoms.

Behavioral therapies focus less on insight. Rather, these approaches try to help a person to change immediate behaviors that contribute to illness or to gain greater satisfaction from routine activities. *Behavioral therapy* and *cognitive-behavioral therapy* concentrate on defining how a person's behaviors affect problems that contribute to depression, then on changing those behaviors. Cognitive-behavioral therapy is particularly useful when patients have negative or distorted attitudes—typically about themselves or the people and events around them—that contribute to depression. Behavioral therapies are useful in treating mild to moderate depression, especially when these therapies are combined with medications.

Marital therapy and *family therapy* combine behavioral, psychodynamic, or interpersonal techniques and educational efforts to address problems that are common among family members in the context of depression. For example, withdrawn or rejecting behaviors by a depressed spouse or parent may be distressing to other members of a family. Interaction styles within a family may increase one member's vulnerability to depression or may hamper the recovery of a patient in treatment.

Group therapy is particularly useful for people who may benefit from sharing observations and insights with other individuals who have depression or other mood disorders. Medication maintenance support groups offer similar benefits; they also provide education about medication and stress the importance of adherence to treatment. Other groups provide information to the patient and family members. The discussion of shared experiences helps to reinforce the message that a mental illness is not different from a general medical illness and can be effectively treated. Groups run by and for patients, such as those of the National Depressive and Manic-Depressive Association (NDMDA), are often useful complements to formal psychotherapy.

Psychotherapy alone is quite effective in treating minor depression. Although psychotherapy alone is rarely adequate for treating moderate or severe depression effectively, it can be an essential part of treatment for such depression. Sessions allow a therapist to monitor the progress of treatment, to provide feedback to a patient about the status of his or her illness, and to discuss any concerns a patient may have about other components of treatment, especially medications. Also, whether the goal of psychotherapy is insight or strategies for immediate behaviors, the process better arms a patient to understand and manage depressions that may arise in the future.

Electroconvulsive Therapy

Electroconvulsive therapy (ECT) is an exceptionally effective treatment for depression. It relieves symptoms quickly, which is particularly useful when an episode of depression involves unmanageable suicidal behaviors or a refusal to eat that could lead to dangerous malnutrition. ECT is also a good alternative treatment when a patient's depression is accompanied by psychotic symptoms, or when use of medication is discouraged (such as during pregnancy).

During ECT the brain is stimulated with an electrical current to produce a seizure. Anesthesia and a muscle relaxant are used to prevent a convulsion in the rest of the body. The chief side effects of ECT are a brief period of confusion following the treatment and temporary memory loss. No medical considerations absolutely prohibit the use of ECT, but for a patient with a recent history of heart attack(s), irregular heart rhythms, or other heart conditions, there is a need for caution. The treatment causes a brief rise in heart rate and blood pressure and causes additional work for the heart.

Unfortunately, because the side effects of ECT and the methods of administering it have been misrepresented and have received negative publicity, there is a stigma attached to this therapy. As it is administered today, however, ECT is very safe, and there is a high level of patient satisfaction with it. In one study, 80% of severely depressed patients who had had ECT expressed willingness to have the treatment again if needed. Moreover, ECT has the highest rate of response of any antidepressant treatment. It should be considered when repeated medication strategies fail. Approximately 50% of patients for whom medications do not work benefit from ECT.

Light Therapy

Seasonal affective disorder is a subtype of depression in which symptoms of the illness appear annually in the late fall, when the days grow shorter, and lessen or disappear in the spring with the return of longer daylight hours. Although the precise cause of the illness is unclear, its responsiveness to treatment strongly suggests a disturbance of brain chemistry.

Light therapy, or *phototherapy,* in which inadequate natural light is supplemented by bright artificial light, is effective in relieving the symptoms of seasonal affective disorder. The lights are specially made to produce the full spectrum of natural light, except for ultraviolet rays. A person with seasonal affective disorder sits by the light for about 30 minutes or more in the morning and possibly again in the evening.

Light therapy alone may relieve symptoms of a mild seasonal affective disorder. At other times, however, light therapy may be used in conjunction with antidepressant medication. No interactions between light therapy and medications are known. Reported side effects such as headache, eyestrain, insomnia, and irritability are relatively minor.

St. John's Wort

St. John's wort (hypericum) is a plant product that has antidepressant properties. Available over the counter, St. John's wort is not regulated as a drug by the Food and Drug Administration; therefore, different preparations may have different ingredients or strengths. Although it is widely used in Germany for the treatment of depression, St. John's wort has not been used or studied as extensively in the United States. It may be comparable to low doses of tricyclic antidepressants for the treatment of mild to moderate depression.

What If Antidepressant Treatment Fails?

For about one in four patients, an initial course of medication does not relieve depression. If this happens, several steps can be taken to identify a treatment program that will work. After 4 to 8 weeks of no response, the doctor should first make sure that the patient is taking the right amount of medication and that no interactions are causing a decrease in the level of medication in the patient's system. Then, the treatment plan can be revised in one of the following ways:

▶ The current medication can be taken for an additional 2 to 4 weeks.

▶ The dose of the current medication can be increased.

▶ Psychotherapy can be added, changed, or increased.

▶ The patient can be switched to a different antidepressant (other than an MAOI).

▶ Other medications can be added to the current medication, including another (non-MAOI) antidepressant, the mood stabilizer lithium, thyroid hormone, an anticonvulsant, or a stimulant.

▶ The patient can be switched to an MAOI.

▶ ECT can be tried.

If a patient is switched from an SSRI to an MAOI, all antidepressant medications should be stopped for several weeks to allow the SSRI to leave, or "wash out of," the patient's system. The washout period avoids the risk of the two medications interacting in a way that might be dangerous. Similarly, if lithium is being taken, it should be stopped before

ECT is performed so that there will be no adverse impact on the ECT-induced seizure.

Any change in treatment should be followed by close monitoring. If there is not at least a moderate improvement in symptoms after an additional 4 to 8 weeks of treatment, the doctor will double-check the information obtained from the initial diagnostic evaluation and review the patient's relevant life circumstances. Any new information obtained from this review can be used to select the next treatment option. When initial treatments fail to work, it can be discouraging to patients, but 80% to 90% of patients with major depressive disorder eventually find a treatment that is effective for them.

Continuation Phase

The various combinations of the treatment approaches just described are quite effective in relieving immediate symptoms of major depressive disorder in a large majority of patients. A note of caution, however: discontinuing treatment for depression too soon after acute symptoms are relieved is likely to result in relapse. The risk of relapse is highest during the first 2 months or so after symptoms disappear.

Generally, a patient who has responded well to antidepressant medication after experiencing a first episode of depression should remain on the full dose of medication for at least 4 to 5 months. Doctor visits during this time can gradually decrease in frequency to every other month for a patient who is stable. For those in active psychotherapy, visits can remain as frequent as 2 to 3 times per week. Psychotherapeutic approaches may be used during the continuation phase. The goal of psychotherapy during this phase is to help patients manage stresses that could increase the likelihood of relapse or that could undermine a patient's intent to follow a prescribed medication plan.

Maintenance Phase

Some patients are particularly prone to recurrence of illness:

▶ People who had dysthymia before their first episode of major depressive disorder or who reverted to dysthymia after treatment; they are likely to have another episode of major depressive disorder

▶ People who have a psychiatric illness, such as an anxiety disorder, in addition to major depressive disorder

▶ Those with a chronic general medical illness

▶ Those who have had a previous major depressive episode

For the last group of patients especially, a long-term program of medication and possibly psychotherapy is recommended to prevent future episodes or to lessen the severity of episodes that do occur. As in the continuation phase, doctor visits may be once or twice a week or only every several months.

A maintenance treatment program can employ the full array of treatments that proved useful in resolving the acute episode of depression. The patient should keep taking medication at the full, effective dose, because lower doses may not provide a preventive effect. Lithium, which is a *mood stabilizer* as opposed to an antidepressant, may also be recommended as a maintenance treatment.

The success of a maintenance medication program will depend on a person's willingness to take medications over a long period of time, possibly for years. If a patient prefers to stop taking medications, they should be tapered off gradually.

If a patient agrees to extended treatment, maintenance psychotherapy may be useful for 1) working on issues of compliance with medication over time or 2) continuing to explore unresolved psychological and interpersonal conflicts. Although psychotherapy does not generally prevent recurrence of depression, therapy may extend the length of well periods between episodes for patients with milder depression who are not taking medications.

Maintenance use of ECT may be a possibility for some people. Candidates for this approach include patients who initially responded well to ECT; those who relapse to a moderate or severe depression while taking antidepressant medications, with or without lithium; and patients who cannot tolerate medications.

Features About the Patient That Influence Treatment

Many features about a patient and his or her life circumstances might suggest a treatment plan and dictate the need to modify or change it as treatment progresses. Features that are particularly important include the risk of suicidal behaviors, psychiatric disorders in addition to major depressive disorder, pregnancy, and general medical illnesses.

Suicide Risk

Although appropriate treatment for major depressive disorder is remarkably effective in preventing suicide, treatment does not eliminate all risk of this very fundamental feature of the illness. The risk of a patient's acting on a suicidal impulse may increase early in treatment. At this point, antidepressant medications have begun to restore a patient's energy and thus ability to take action, but the depressive mood and sense of hopelessness common to depression have not yet gone away.

Other Psychiatric Disorders

Major depressive disorder is often complicated by patients' having another psychiatric illness as well, such as a substance (drug or alcohol) abuse or dependence disorder, panic or other anxiety disorders, or a personality disorder. Treating and managing these combined or overlapping conditions can be very challenging. Fortunately, newer medications and a better understanding of the properties of older medications offer treatment opportunities that did not exist only a few years ago. Certain of the SSRIs, for example, and the cyclic antidepressant clomipramine are effective in treating depressive disorders as well as obsessive-compulsive disorder. The cyclic antidepressant amoxapine is effective in treating depression with psychotic features. Another choice of treatment for depression with psychotic features is an antidepressant and an antipsychotic medication together. A patient should discuss the pros and cons of these various approaches with his or her doctor.

Patients with both substance abuse and depressive illness are more likely to attempt suicide and less likely to comply with treatment. Achieving sobriety is an urgent first task in treating depression in these patients. As noted previously, achieving sobriety may require hospitalization. There is a risk of dangerous interactions between psychiatric medication and other drugs that a patient is using. Therefore, such patients must have careful medical monitoring, including blood testing.

In older patients, many symptoms that once would have been interpreted as signaling a degenerative brain disease or dementia can actually be traced to depression. These patients are easily helped by treatment. The most telling symptoms are those involving memory, ability to concentrate, and interest in self-care. Antidepressant medications and ECT are highly effective for people whose depression shows these symptoms.

Pregnancy

Although women with major depressive disorder certainly can have successful pregnancies, they should be aware of risks associated with the use of antidepressant and other psychiatric medications during pregnancy and, if possible, discuss any plans for pregnancy with their psychiatrist. The first trimester is the period of highest risk for the fetus. In the other phases of pregnancy, medications can be used if warranted for the mother's well-being. If use of medications is not feasible, ECT is a safe procedure for mother and fetus.

A woman who stops maintenance antidepressant treatment during pregnancy may be at high risk for recurrence of depression. She should have medications restored promptly after the baby is born. A psychiatrist will advise a mother of the risks and benefits that must be balanced in making a decision about nursing a newborn while the mother is taking antidepressants or lithium, given the chance that chemicals from the medication will pass to the child.

General Medical Conditions

People with certain chronic physical illnesses not only can become depressed; they may also be at higher than average risk for major depressive disorder. The presence of some conditions may complicate treatment with certain antidepressant medications, because the side effects of the antidepressant medication may worsen the physical illness. This is true for asthma, cardiac disease, dementia, epilepsy, glaucoma, high blood pressure, obstructive kidney and bladder disease, and Parkinson's disease. At the same time, because there are so many different antidepressant medications now available, there are safe choices in most situations.

Before developing a treatment plan that involves use of medication, a psychiatrist must be fully aware of all medications that a patient is taking for other purposes. In some instances, the psychiatrist may consult directly with other specialists who are treating the patient. For example, in the treatment of a patient with heart disease, the psychiatrist may consult with the cardiologist.

When antidepressant medications cannot be taken by a patient with a general medical condition, ECT is often an appropriate, effective treatment for depression. In some illnesses, such as epilepsy and Parkinson's disease, ECT may offer temporary relief of nonpsychiatric symptoms as well. It is important for all physicians and other members of the health care team who are involved in a patient's care to be fully informed of the various factors that influence a patient's health.

Sources of Additional Information

American Psychiatric Association
1400 K Street, N.W.
Washington, DC 20005
Telephone: 888-35-PSYCH (888-357-7924)
Web: www.psych.org

Internet Mental Health
Web: www.mentalhealth.com

National Alliance for the Mentally Ill (NAMI)
Colonial Place Three
2107 Wilson Boulevard, Suite 300
Arlington, VA 22201-3042
Telephone: 800-950-NAMI (800-950-6264)
    (speak with an individual on HELPLINE, Monday–Friday,
    10:00 A.M.–5:00 P.M. Eastern Time; message line, any other time)
Web: www.nami.org

National Depressive and Manic-Depressive Association
730 North Franklin Street, Suite 501
Chicago, IL 60610
Telephone: 800-826-3632
Web: www.ndmda.org

National Foundation for Depressive Illness
P.O. Box 2257
New York, NY 10116
Telephone: 800-239-1265
Web: www.depression.org

National Institute of Mental Health
Depression Information Program
6001 Executive Boulevard, Room 8184, MSC 9663
Bethesda, MD 20892-9663
Telephone: 800-421-4211 (to request free printed information)
    Or 301-443-4513 (to speak with an information specialist)
Web: www.nimh.nih.gov

National Mental Health Association
1021 Prince Street
Alexandria, VA 22314-2971
Telephone: 800-969-NMHA (800-969-6642)
    Or 703-684-7722
Web: www.nmha.org

www.ingramcontent.com/pod-product-compliance
Ingram Content Group UK Ltd.
Pitfield, Milton Keynes, MK11 3LW, UK
UKHW021834140426
5217IPUK00021B/1441